Thorsons First Directions

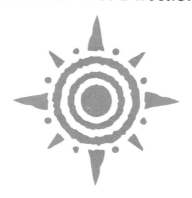

Indian Head Massage

Narendra Mehta

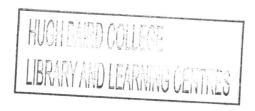

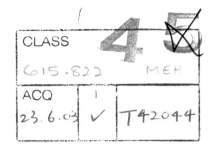
Thorsons
An Imprint of HarperCollins*Publishers*
77–85 Fulham Palace Road,
Hammersmith, London W6 8JB

The Thorsons website address is:
www.thorsons.com

Published by Thorsons 2001
Text derived from *Indian Head Massage: discover the power of touch* published
by Thorsons 1999

10 9 8 7 6 5 4 3 2 1

Editor: Susan Bosanko
Design: Wheelhouse Creative
Photography: Simon McComb
Production: Melanie Vandevelde
Text illustration: Jane Spencer

A catalogue record for this book is available from the British Library

ISBN 0 00 712356 6

Printed and bound in Hong Kong

Narendra Mehta's London Centre of Indian Champissage is at the Eastern Health and Beauty
Centre, 136 Holloway Road, London N7 8DD, telephone 020 7609 3590, fax 020 7607 4228

Contents

Indian Head Massage

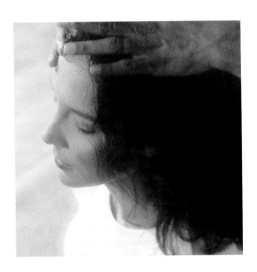

dispels stress, relieves tension in the neck, head a

oulders, and promotes healthy hair

What is Indian Head Massage?

Indian head massage is a safe, simple, yet effective therapy that not only promotes hair growth, but also provides relief from aches and pains. It is renowned for relieving symptoms of stress.

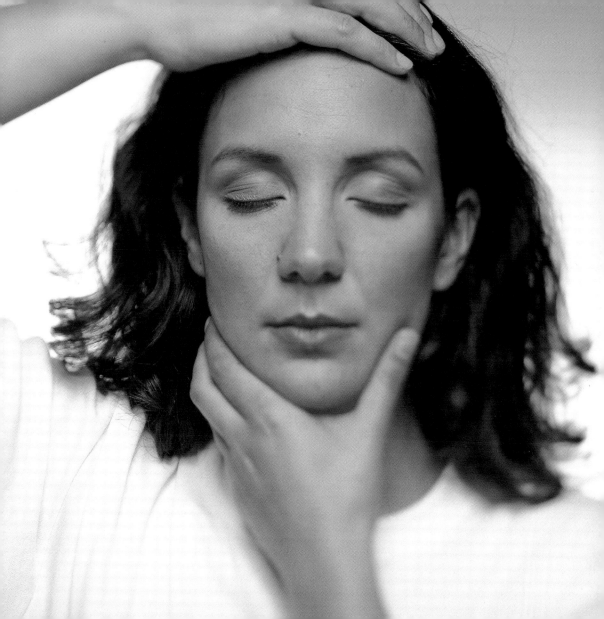

History

Massage has always played an important part in Indian life. When used in conjunction with herbs, spices and aromatic oils, massage had an important medical function and could not only 'strengthen muscles and firm the skin' but also encourage the body's natural healing abilities. Today, Indian infants still often receive a daily massage from birth to keep them in good health. From three to six years old, they are massaged once or twice a week, and after the age of six, they are taught to share a massage with family members on a regular basis. Massage then occurs across the generations as an integral and natural part of family life.

Indian head massage springs from this rich tradition of intergenerational family massage, and has been practised for over a thousand years. It was originally developed by women as part of their grooming routine. They used different oils according to the season to keep their hair strong, lustrous and in beautiful condition.

The benefits of head massage were not confined exclusively to women: barbers practised many of these same skills. They used to ply their

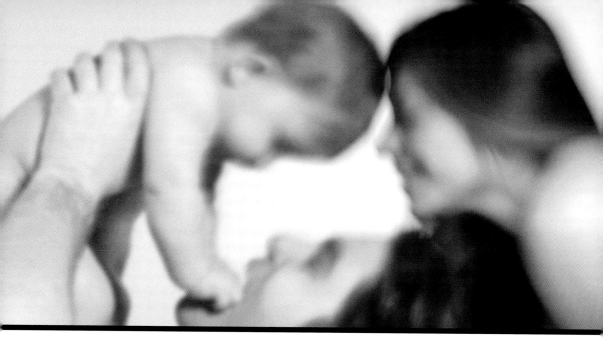

trade by going to individuals' houses, cutting men's hair and offering 'champi' (head massage) as part of the treatment. In time, this became quite a custom: everyone, including royalty, would receive regular head massage from their own barber. Treatments differed from the massages performed by women in that the barbers were mainly giving invigorating scalp massages designed primarily to stimulate and refresh the individual, rather than to care for the hair. Echoes of this Indian tradition reached the West long before the practice itself in the form of the word 'shampoo', which comes from the Hindi word 'champi'. Being 'champi-ed' meant having your head massaged.

Massage skills have evolved through the ages and have been handed down from barber father to barber son in much the same way that the women in the family have kept the tradition of hair massage and grooming by passing it down from mother to daughter right up to the present day.

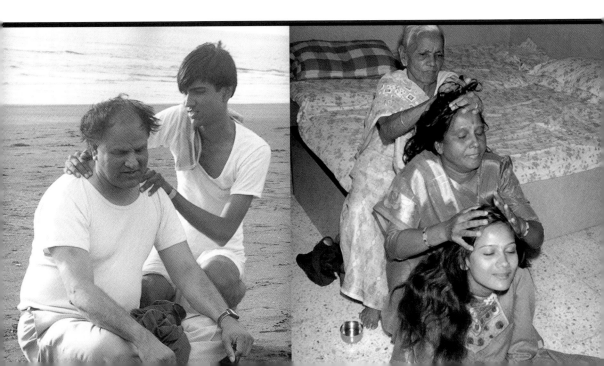

Development

Like most of my compatriots, I grew up with head massage as an integral part of my daily life. As a child, my mother would give me a head massage and, as I grew older, it was something to be automatically experienced every time I visited a barber.

When I came to England to study, I began to miss the therapeutic value of regular head massage and decided that I wanted to bring this therapy to the West. Experience had taught me that head massage could bring tremendous relief from aches and pains, not only in the head, but also in other parts of the body. After much research in India, I developed and formalized a therapy that would bring the greatest relief to the multitude of problems concentrated in the head. I soon concluded that the therapy would benefit by being extended to include not only the head, but also the neck, shoulders and upper arms.

Since then I have been passing on my knowledge at my clinic, at exhibitions, and through courses. Now you can learn these techniques, which combine an ancient cultural tradition with the demands of modern living, to use at home.

How does it work?

The head, neck and shoulders are important energy centres within your body. If you are feeling stressed or angry, tension tends to accumulate. The tension can later show up as a stiff neck and shoulders, as eye strain and sometimes even as hair loss. Indian head massage involves working with a firm and gentle rhythm to help unknot blockages and relieve this uncomfortable build-up of tension. However, its effect is not just physical: it works on an emotional level too, calming the spirit, promoting relaxation and relieving stress. It tackles the physical, mental and emotional effects of stress in a unique and particularly effective way.

As the head, face and neck store a great deal of the anxiety, emotion and tension that accumulates in everyday life, touching these areas through massage will help to melt away troubles and open the paths of communication and understanding. If people massaged each other's head and hair on a regular basis, the world would be a happier and more loving place. The head and hair are extremely sensitive as the face and scalp are crowded with nerve endings. This makes them extremely receptive to touch. Massaging the head and hair is soothing and deeply relaxing.

The Benefits of Indian Head Massage

The power of touch

Touch is essential for stimulating our nervous system and promoting healthy physical development. It is also critical for our mental and social development.

As babies, our most powerful experiences come through the medium of touch. We reach out to touch and explore the world around us, and we are also held and cradled by our parents. A large part of the way we feel about ourselves comes from the way we are held and touched by our parents.

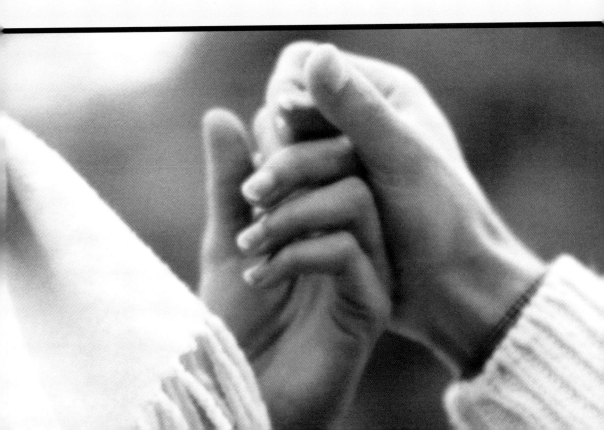

We learn about pleasure, warmth and comfort from touch. We learn about expressing our feelings, we learn about reassurance and security, and we learn about connectedness and social bonding. Touch connects us to the outside world, brings people closer and weaves intimacy.

Touch is an instinctive, natural language that we all speak and understand. It is from this instinctive language that more structured forms of touch have evolved to eventually develop into the different forms of massage that exist in every culture throughout the world. One of the wonderful things about massage is that it is a formalized touch: it gives you permission to touch someone within established and defined boundaries. A particular benefit of Indian head massage is that you do not need to undress to be treated, and so it can be practised anywhere, at any time.

Massage is a wonderful way to share time and emotion and the power of touch with your partner. It can soothe tension and misunderstanding and reinforce feelings of tenderness and intimacy. Together you can participate in a cycle of mutual giving and receiving.

Skin and hair

Massage helps to drain away the toxins that gather in your skin and muscles, and it improves your circulation. Regular sessions can help to improve the texture and tone of your skin, leaving it noticeably silkier and smoother.

Massaging the head helps to spread the natural oils produced by the scalp along the whole length of the hair, allowing them to protect and condition right to the tips.

Massaging the scalp improves the circulation, helping to nourish the hair from the roots and drain away any toxins that may accumulate. A regular massage will keep your scalp in tip top condition and help your hair to feel thicker and shinier.

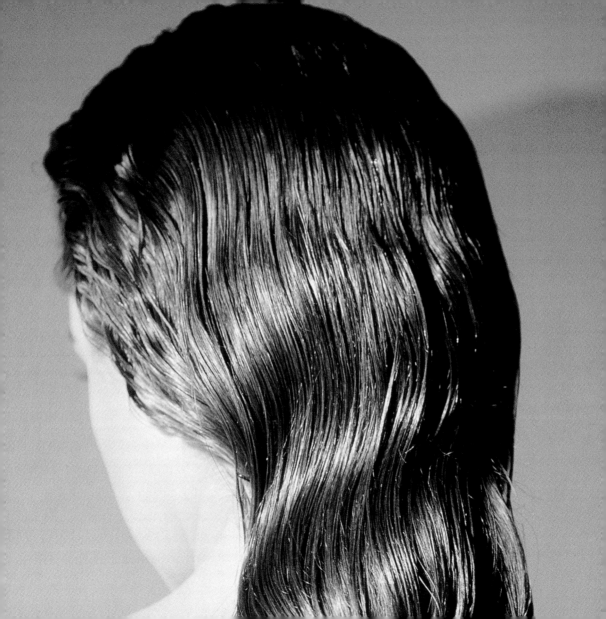

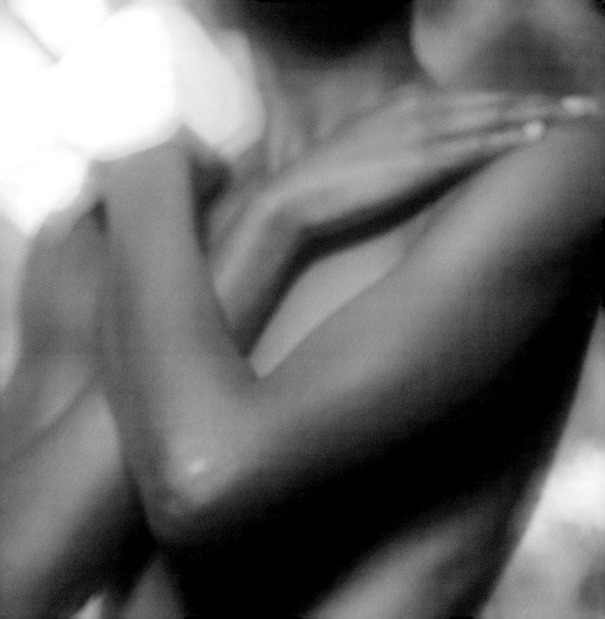

Muscular strains
and headaches

The shoulder area is one of the most common areas of tension, stiffness and loss of flexibility. Indian head massage not only relaxes the muscles in this area, restoring joint movement in the neck and shoulders, but also stimulates the blood and lymphatic system to help eliminate toxins and speed healing.

The back of the neck contains a complex network of muscles and nerves and so is particularly vulnerable to tension and strains. Indian head massage is excellent for relieving stiff, sore neck muscles and minor strains.

Headaches caused by stress and tension seem to be an inevitable part of modern life. Painkillers may block the 'pain messages' and relieve the pain, but massage tackles the problem at its source – relaxing the tense muscles that cause the problem.

Other benefits

Indian head massage provides a de-stressing programme for the whole body and has a far-reaching effect on every one of the body's systems. It can provide help for mental tiredness and edginess, relieve emotional stress, improve concentration, promote relaxation, and is excellent for disturbed sleep and insomnia.

An exhaustive list of its benefits is impossible, as everyone who has experienced it will want to add their own suggestions.

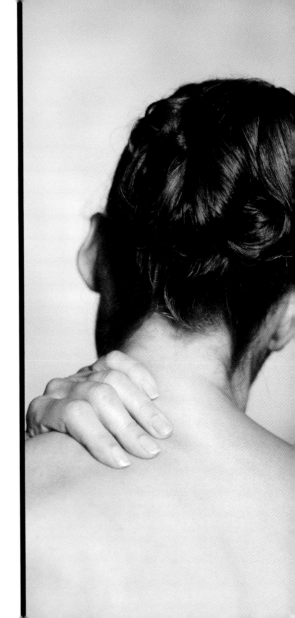

Basic Massage Techniques

To gain the maximum benefit, each technique should be repeated three times.

Throughout this book you will find movements described as 'friction' or 'rubbing': so what's the difference? Friction requires fairly heavy pressure and should cause the skin to move over the bones of the scalp with your hand. A rub is a lighter motion: your hand should move over the surface of the skin.

You do not need to use any oils or creams during a massage unless you choose to do so (in which case, see the section on Using Oils).

Words of caution

Indian head massage is very easy to use, but it must be treated with respect and the instructions followed carefully, if they are to be safe and effective. You should not practise Indian head massage on anyone who is currently suffering from any chronic or acute health problems, or who is undergoing medical treatment for any serious conditions, or who is drunk. Indian head massage is a very safe and beneficial therapy, but it is not intended to be a substitute for medical treatment.

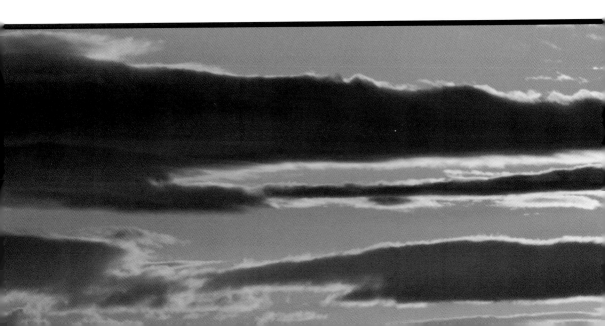

First things first

Ask the person who is receiving the massage to remove any neck-chains, earrings or other jewellery, or spectacles. If they want to remove their shoes they can do so.

Ask them to sit down in an upright chair where you will feel comfortable massaging them without having to tense your own arms and shoulders. When they are seated, make sure they do not have their

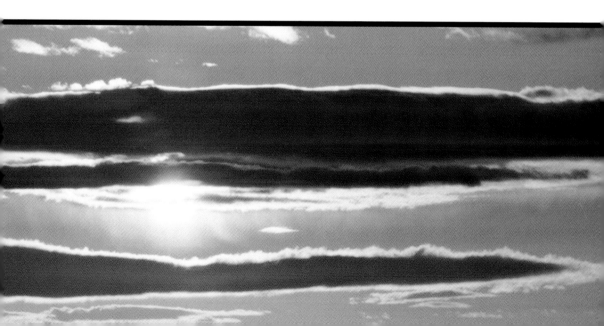

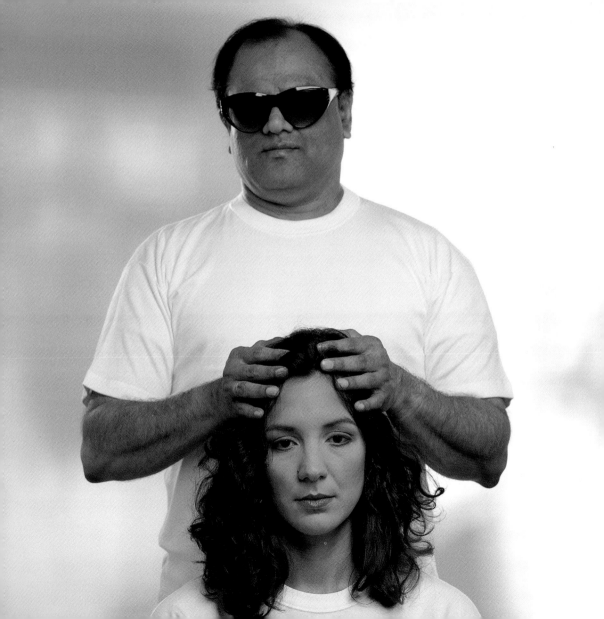

knees crossed or their feet crossed at the ankles. Ask them to place the soles of their feet firmly on the ground and to place their hands in a relaxed position in their lap.

Stand behind them and lay your hands very lightly on the top of their head. Remember to make sure that your hands and nails are clean and that your hands are warm – cold hands on the head will certainly not help induce a state of relaxation. If necessary, run your hands under hot water to warm them up.

Relax. Now ask the person receiving the massage to relax and do a simple breathing exercise with you. Close your mouth and breathe in and out, deeply and gently, three times through your nostrils.

Both of you will become more grounded and in touch if you use this simple technique before every massage. It relaxes you and stills your mind, concentrating your energy on the task in hand.

If you are going to use oil in your massage, apply it now (see the section on Using Oils for further information).

Shoulder and upper arm massage

Thumb push

Place the palms of your hands at the corners of the shoulders with thumbs resting above the shoulder blades. Push with your thumbs, using medium pressure, up and over the shoulder muscles. Now pull back the muscles, dragging your fingers towards your thumbs, using medium pressure. Repeat the action at the middle of the shoulders, then again at the junction of the neck and shoulders.

By applying pressure on the shoulder muscles, you are helping to break down knots and nodules. In effect, you are squeezing out toxins and softening up the muscles.

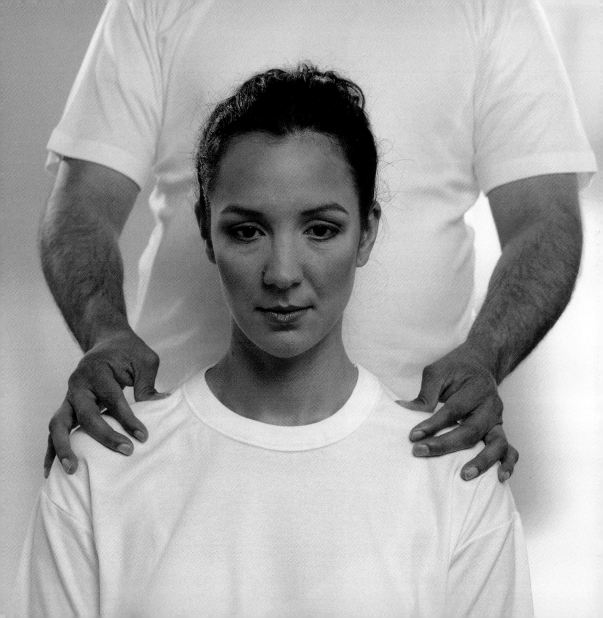

Heel push

In some cases, you may not be able to do the thumb push because the shoulders are too broad. In this case, you can use the heels of your hands instead of your thumbs. This has exactly the same effect as the thumb push, but allows you to exert more pressure while you work the same area without becoming tired.

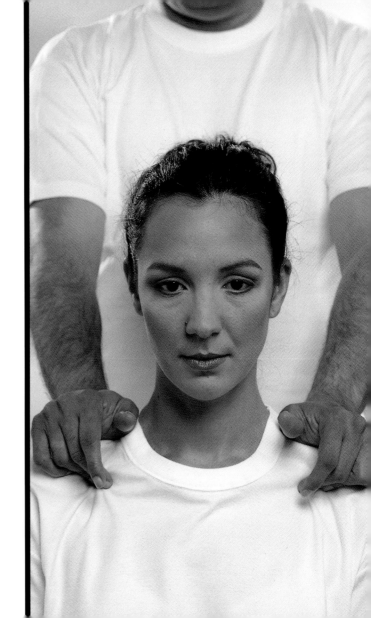

Finger pulls

Place your thumbs between the shoulder blades and your fingers near the neck in front of the shoulder muscles. Pull back the muscles, dragging your fingers towards your thumbs, using medium pressure. Repeat at the middle of the shoulders, and again further along the muscles near the corner of the shoulders.

By applying pressure on the shoulder muscles, you are helping to break down knots and nodules. In effect, you are squeezing out toxins and softening up the muscles.

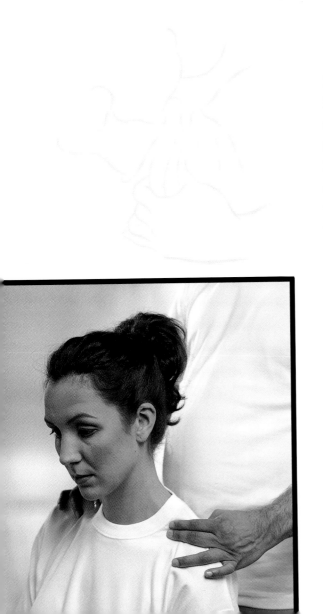

Pick up and squeeze

Place the palms of your hands on the corners of the shoulders with your thumbs behind the shoulder muscles and your fingers in front. Push your thumbs towards your fingers, gathering as much muscle as possible. Squeeze using medium pressure and hold for a few seconds, then let go. Repeat at the middle of the shoulders. Repeat near the neck.

This technique helps to squeeze out toxins from the tight muscles, making them softer and more mobile. It also helps to break down fibrous adhesions.

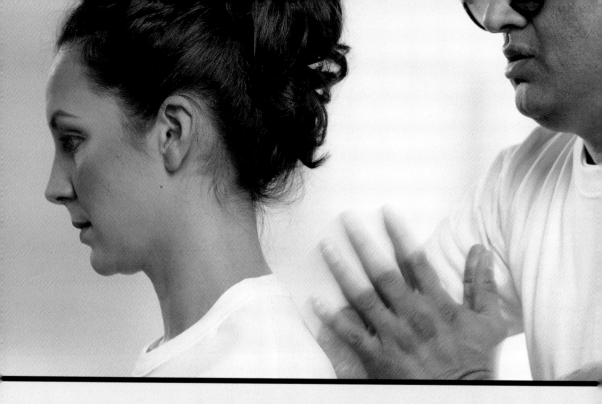

Champi

Place your hands together in a prayer position, keeping your wrists relaxed. Make quick, light hitting movements with your little fingers across the shoulders, touching the muscles only.

This technique will stimulate the blood circulation.

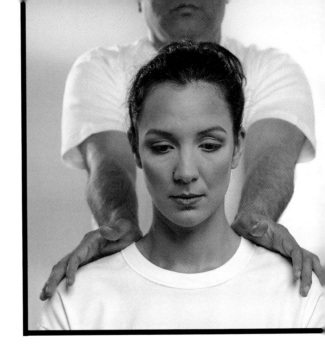

Ironing down

Place the heels of your hands on either side of the neck. Point your fingers towards the corners of the shoulders. Apply medium pressure and slide both hands across the shoulder muscles to the edge of the shoulder.

This helps to drain away toxins and bring the shoulders down, and is a superb muscle relaxer.

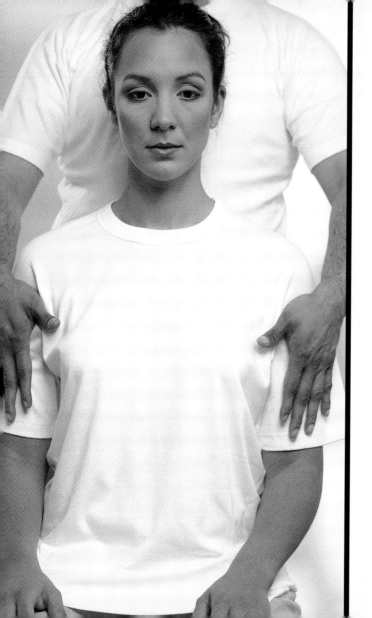

Ironing down the shoulders leads naturally on to working with the upper arms: continue the movement with the heels of your hands to relax and loosen the arm muscles. Work from the top of the arm down to the elbow, using firm pressure. Go down the sides of the arms, and then down the front of the arms.

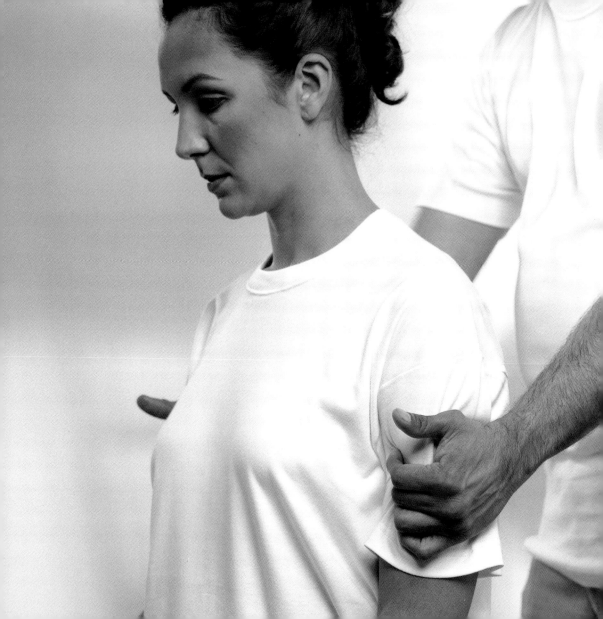

Heel roll

Place your hands on the top of the arms (on the deltoid muscles), fingers in front, heels behind. With firm pressure, roll the heels of your hands forwards over the muscles to arrive at your fingertips. Repeat at the middle of the upper arm, then again just above the elbow. Make sure that you do not pinch the muscles at the end of the stroke and so spoil the effect.

Neck massage

Grasp and pull back

With one hand on the forehead, tilt the neck back slightly. With the other hand, spread your thumb and fingers as far as possible on either side of the base of the neck. Using medium pressure, slide your hand up to the top of the neck, grasp the flesh and pull it back. Grasp at the middle of the neck and pull back, and then grasp at the base of the neck and pull back.

This is a soft tissue mobilization technique that loosens up the neck muscles.

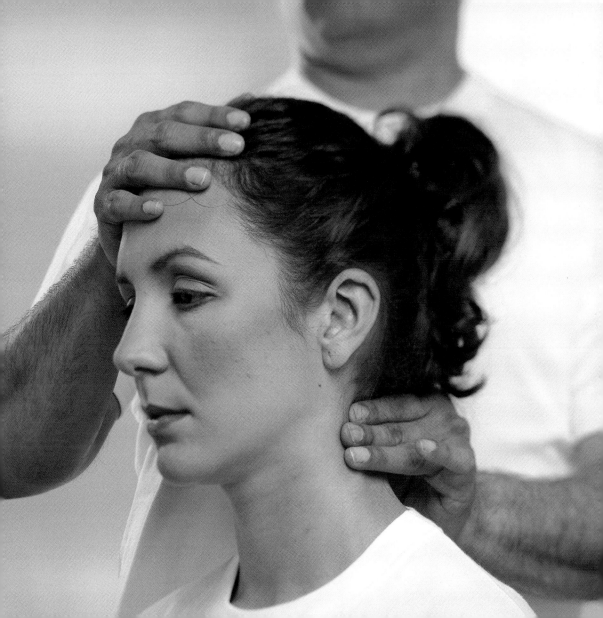

Friction under the occiput

Warm up the muscles under the occiput (base of the skull) by using your fingertips to create gentle friction at the base of the skull. Support the forehead and work your way back and forth from behind the ear to the top of the spine. Repeat this on the other side of the head.

This technique helps to loosen up congested muscles and releases toxins to be drained away.

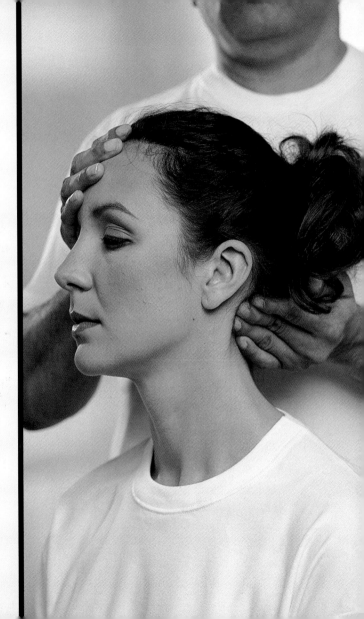

Heel rub under the occiput

Place your right hand over the front of the forehead to support the head, then tilt the head forwards just slightly. Place the heel of your left hand against the base of the skull (occiput) and rub lightly and briskly over the surface of the skin.

This stimulates the circulation and drains toxins away. It is an excellent technique for relieving the pain of strained muscles in the neck.

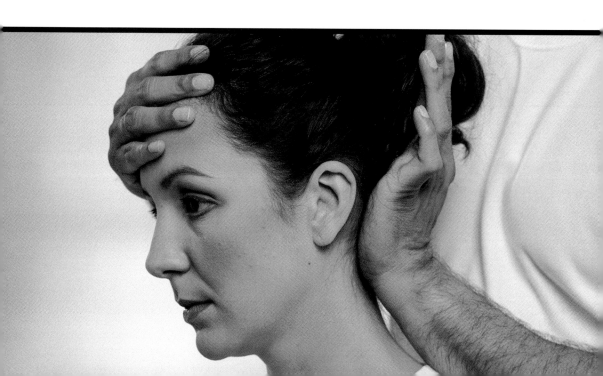

Scalp massage

Windscreen wiper

Place your hand in front of the ear with your fingers on the forehead to support the head. Following the given route, use the ball of the other hand to carry out a light rubbing movement on the other side of the head. Repeat this on the opposite side of the head, then repeat twice more on both sides.

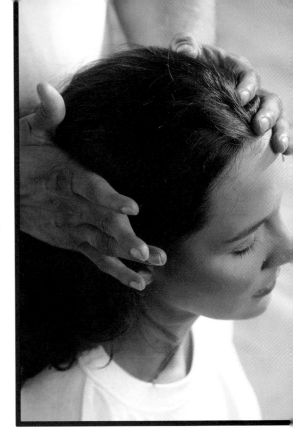

This movement is designed to warm up and stimulate the scalp, improving its overall condition.

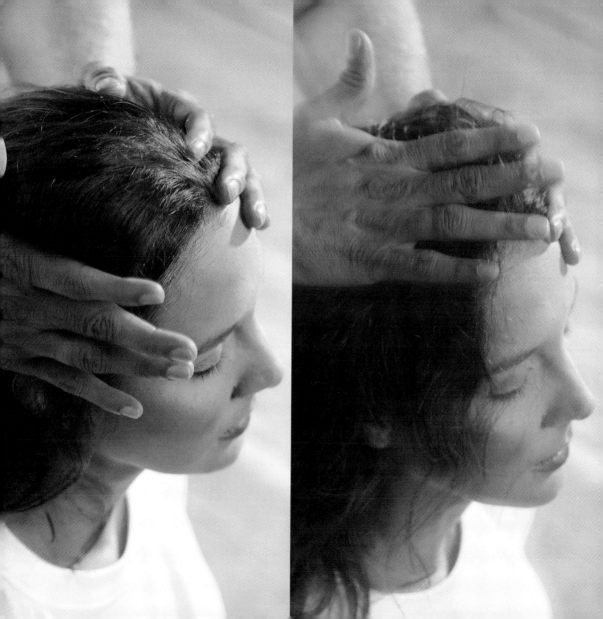

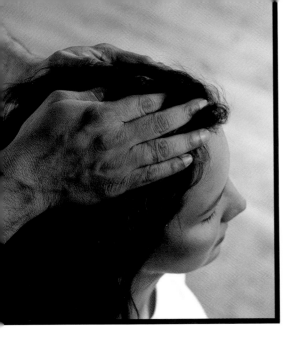

Whole hand friction

This is a friction movement and not a rub, so do not allow your hands to slide over the scalp – the scalp should move under your hand.

Place both hands above the ears with your fingers pointing forwards. While the head is supported by one hand, apply firm pressure with the whole of the other hand, including your fingertips and the heel. Move the scalp up and down. Move the hand to a new position slightly above the previous one. Repeat the same action. Repeat the sequence on the other side of the head.

This movement loosens up the tight subcutaneous scalp muscles.

Ruffling

Open the fingers of one hand and, keeping your wrist relaxed and supporting the head with your other hand, lightly ruffle the entire head of hair.

Most people really enjoy this. The lighter the touch, the better. Remember to keep your wrist loose.

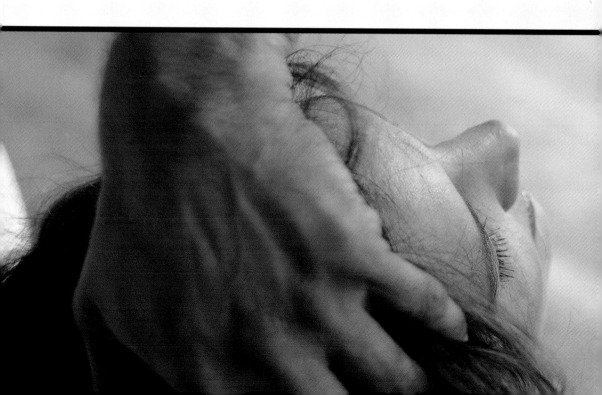

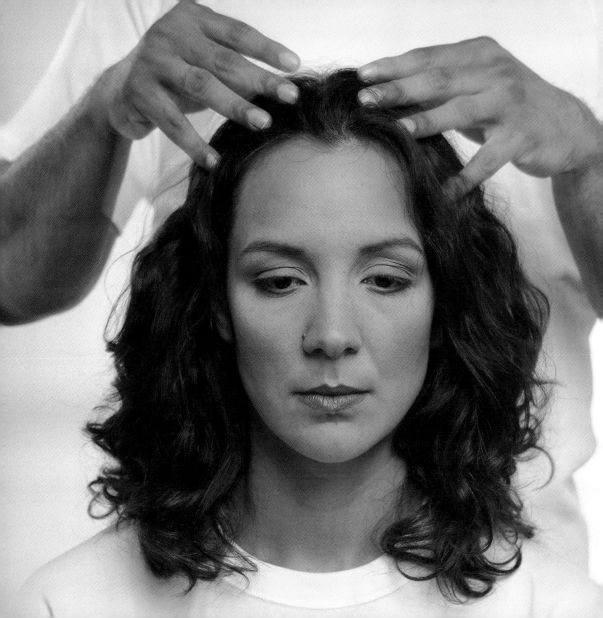

Plucking

Soft landing, quick take off! With your fingers outstretched, land softly on the head. On making contact, spring off, bringing your fingers and thumbs together. Land in a different position, with your fingers again outstretched. Repeat this energetic movement until you have covered the top of the head.

This is a stimulating technique that brings the circulation to the surface.

Stroking

Place one hand flat over the top of the head with the fingers pointing forwards at the beginning of the hairline, and gently bring the hand towards the back of the head. Follow with the other hand so that a wave-like continuity is established and the person receiving the massage is unaware of where one stroke begins and another finishes.

Use a similar stroking action while running your fingers and the fingernails of both hands through the hair, creating the same wave-like continuity.

Both these stroking techniques will intensify the feelings of relaxation, remove any feelings of stress, and make the other person feel calm and nurtured.

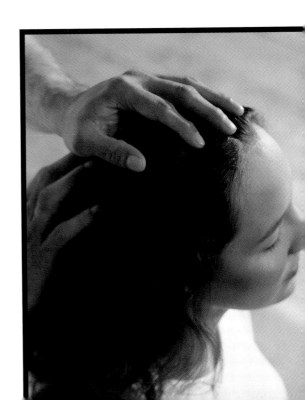

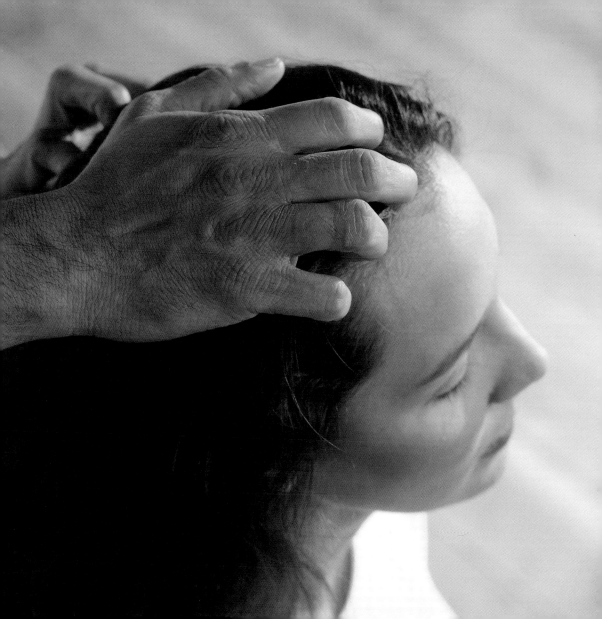

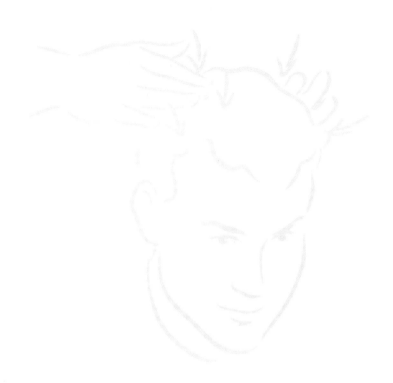

Tabla playing

Use your fingertips to gently tap on the scalp. Imagine that you are playing the piano (or the Indian tabla). Do this until your have covered the entire head.

This technique stimulates the circulation and is surprisingly energizing.

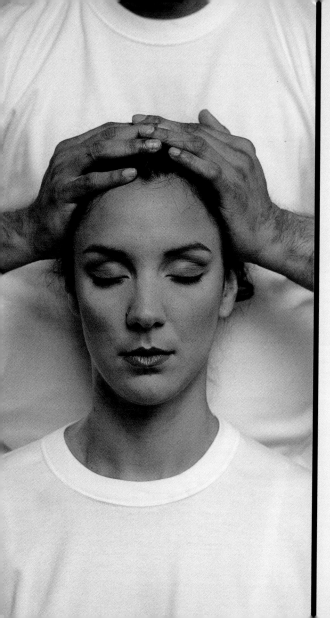

Squeeze and lift

Place your fingertips on top of the head with the heels of your hands behind the ears. Keep your elbows out at right angles. Squeeze inwards with the heels using medium pressure, then lift the scalp with the heels of your hands. Hold for three seconds and then let go. Repeat with the heels of the hands above the ears and then in front of the ears.

This movement is excellent for releasing tension headaches.

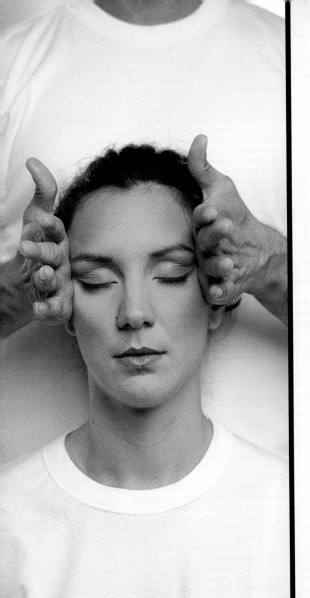

Circular temple friction

Stand close to the person you are massaging and support their head with your body. Make sure that you do not tilt the head too far back as this could be very uncomfortable for the other person.

Place the heels of your hands in front of the ears and the palms over the temples. Use the palms of your hands to make slow, wide, circular movements. Remember this is a friction movement, so the skin should move under your hands.

This movement is excellent for tension headaches in the temple area and wonderful for relieving eyestrain.

Relax the face

Lay your hands on the face with the palms of your hands over the cheeks, then gently trail your fingers up and down the face, giving the warmth of your healing hands. Repeat this movement several times.

We all have healing hands, whether we realize it or not: some people know how to use them and some don't. When you lay your hands on someone's face or head concentrate on sharing your healing energy and feeling the power flowing through your fingertips. All you need to do is to visualize it to make it happen.

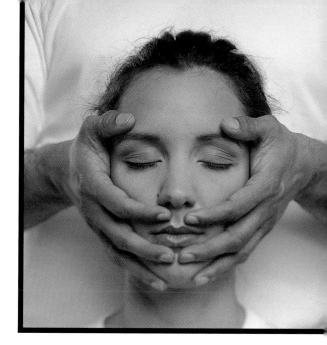

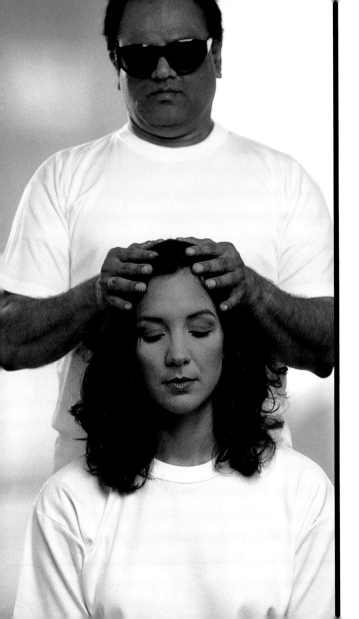

Final scalp massage

Use your imagination! Combine some of the moves that you know the other person especially likes. Be gentle: they may be asleep! Finish off your Indian head massage with some wonderfully relaxing stroking movements. Finally, when you are ready to end the massage, lay your hands again on the other person's head in the same way as you did when you began.

Partners and Lovers

Indian head massage creates a special bond between you and your partner or lover that will bring you closer. A caring massage creates feelings of trust and joy and connects you with your partner on a deep physical, spiritual and emotional level. If you and your partner take time to massage each other regularly, your bodies will become more sensual and receptive, and you will feel more deeply in tune with each other. You may want to work on your partner's bare skin for this massage, and to use aromatherapy oils to heighten the erotic effect.

This massage should be featherlight and rhythmic. The gentle, repetitive moves will release your partner from the day's stress. You, your hands and your imagination will seduce your partner into the most magnificent of mellow, loving moods.

Setting the scene

It is important to set the scene before you start. This will help to relax you both. First, find a draught-free, pleasantly warm room where you know you will not be disturbed – lock the door if necessary. Think about where your partner is going to sit, and make him or her as comfortable as possible. With a bit of imagination rugs, throws, drapes and cushions can transform an ordinary room into an exotic sanctuary. Add some flowers to delight your lover's eye.

Soft lighting will impart a feeling of serenity and peace, so dim the lights: avoid overhead lights and use sidelights or, if possible, candles to create an atmosphere that will soothe and relax. You could also put on some soft, soothing music that both of you like – you don't have to perform the massage in silence. Choose some essential oils to burn in an oil burner to create a subtle fragrance in the room: above all else, fragrance will assist in creating a sensual ambience.

Getting started

You will find more detailed information on the techniques used here in the section on Basic Massage, and on choosing and applying oils in the section on Using Oils. Having clean, warm hands, being relaxed, comfortable and grounded, and establishing a connection with your partner through the simple breathing exercise are particularly important when you are sharing a sensual massage.

Before you apply the oil, try a few warm-up moves. Tell your partner to close their eyes and let their imagination run wild while you begin by stroking their hair, head and face. Don't forget the ears, which are sensual areas: touching them gently helps your partner to get into a really loving mood. Your hands should feel like waves, with no sensation of strokes beginning or ending. For a dramatic change of focus, continue stroking but this time use your fingernails to stroke the hair down the neck and continue down your partner's back. This will make your partner feel fantastic.

You are now ready to apply your chosen oil and to begin this loving and sensual version of Indian head massage.

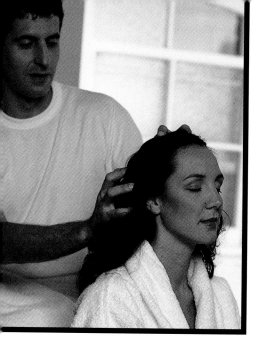

Sensual massage

Stroking

Using both hands, one after another, gently stroke from the front to the back of the head, using long sweeping movements with the whole of the hands. Use very light pressure. This should be followed by running your fingernails through the hair, then down the neck and back. Work all around the head. This action relaxes the scalp and stimulates the circulation, giving your partner a lovely tingly feeling.

Rubbing the back

With the whole of your hand, rub briskly all over the back, using light pressure. This will warm your partner's back and relax him or her.

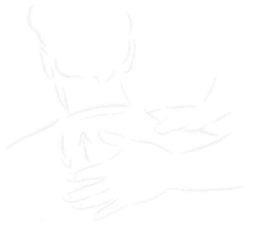

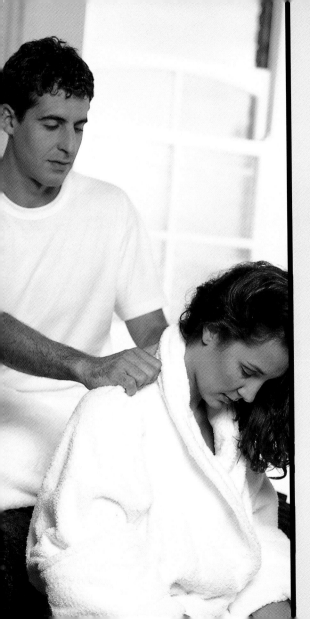

Heel roll on the shoulders

Place the thumb or heel of your hand just above the corner of the shoulder. Roll your thumb or heel forwards, using medium pressure, up and over the shoulder muscles. Repeat at the middle of the shoulders, then again at the junction of the neck and shoulders.

This will help to increase circulation and relieve stress and tension in your partner's shoulders. Use the heel of your hand, rather than the thumb, when your partner's shoulders are broad. This will allow you to exert more pressure over a wider area without getting tired.

Heel squeeze on the shoulders

Reach from one side of your partner across to their other shoulder, placing one of your arms across their front and the other across their back. Squeeze their shoulder muscle with the heels of your hands using medium pressure. Do this in several places along the shoulder. Repeat a few times. This will soften tight muscles and release toxins.

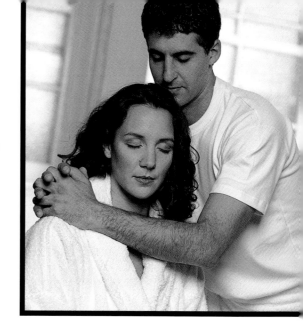

Champi across the shoulders

Place your hands together in a prayer position, keeping your wrists relaxed. Make quick, light hitting movements with your little fingers across the shoulders, touching the muscles only. This will stimulate the blood circulation.

Ironing down

Iron down the upper arms, using the heel of your hand to relax and loosen the arm muscles. Work from the top of the arm down to the elbow using the palms and heels of your hands with medium to deep pressure. Go down the sides of the arms, then down the front and back of the arms. Repeat twice more.

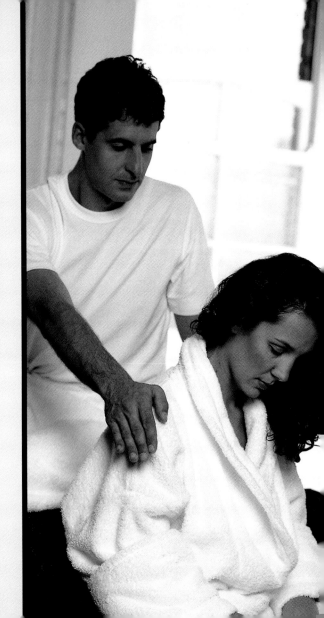

Heel roll

Place your hands on top of the arm over the deltoid muscles. Place your fingers in front and the heels of your hands behind. Roll your heels over the muscles to arrive at your fingertips. Repeat at the middle of the upper arm, and then at just above the elbow.

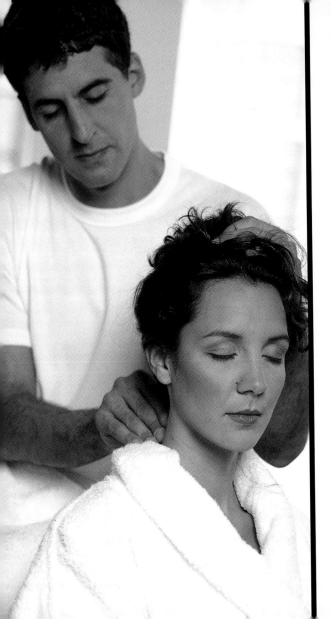

Neck massage

With one hand on the top of
the head, tilt the head
slightly back and with the
other hand spread your
thumb and fingers across the
base of your partner's neck.
Using firm contact with the
skin, slide your hands up the
neck, grasp the flesh and pull
back. Grasp at the middle of
the neck and pull back.
Finally, grasp at the base of
the neck and pull back.
Repeat this a few more times.

This is a soft tissue
mobilization move, which
loosens up the neck muscles.

Heel rub under the back of the head

With one hand supporting the forehead, place the heel of the other hand under the back of the head, pushing the fingers through the hair. Rub quickly and lightly up and down right across the back of the head. This helps to relieve tension in the muscles at the top of the neck and can often relieve tension headaches.

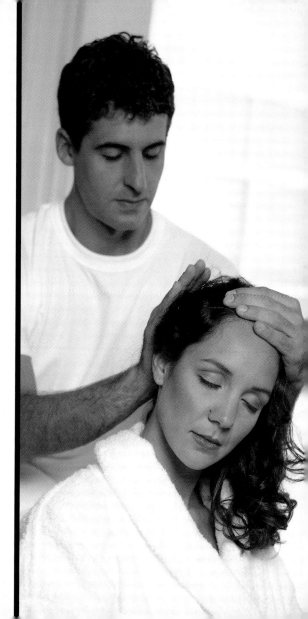

Scalp rub

Support your partner's head with one hand and, using the palm of the other hand, carry out a swift, gentle rubbing movement as if you were washing a window. Start behind the ear, go around it and then away from the ear and up to the top of the head. Repeat the movement on the other side of the head. This relaxes and warms the scalp.

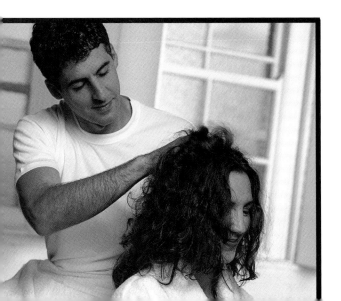

Hair ruffling

Taking the hair between your fingers, ruffle the hair all over the head. This creates a very pleasing sensation.

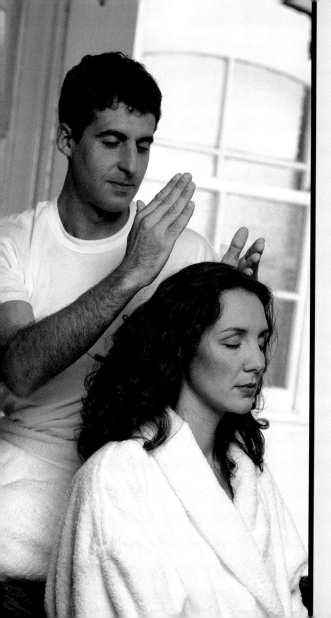

Hacking on the head

Hold both hands over your partner's head, fingers facing forwards and palms facing inwards. Use the fingers of alternate hands to make quick, light hitting movements over the top of the head. Continue for a few minutes, making sure that you cover the whole area of the head.

This pleasantly stimulating technique boosts the circulation and will leave your partner feeling relaxed and refreshed.

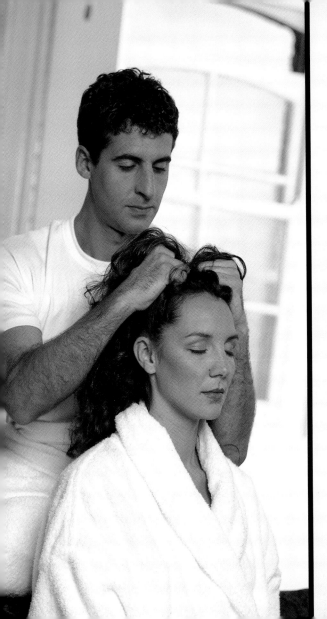

Gathering and tugging the hair

Push your fingers through the hair on either side of your partner's head. Start either at the base of the head or the top of the head. Curl your fingers round into fists, keeping the back of your fingers against the scalp and getting hold of as much hair as you can. Gently tug on the hair. Continue all over the head. If your partner has short hair, then approach this from the top, grasping as much hair as possible. Continue in this way until you have covered the whole head.

Head squeeze and lift

Place the heels of both your hands just above your partner's ears, letting your fingers drop on to the top of the head like a cap. Squeeze with the heels, applying medium pressure, then lift the scalp and hold for a couple of seconds before letting go. Repeat the same move slightly in front of the ears. You can repeat it two or three times. This will help to relieve most headaches and it has a calming effect.

Stroking

Repeat the stroking actions with which you began this sensual massage, working all round the head, giving your partner a lovely tingly feeling.

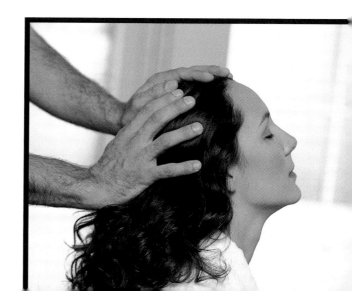

Ear massage

Your ears contain a high concentration of nerve endings and are especially sensitive. Nibbling on your lover's ear is a well-known trick, but ear massage is particularly sensual and will give your partner a wonderful feeling.

Position yourself either directly behind or in front of your partner. Place your flattened palms on your partner's ears and cover them entirely. Rub your flattened palms up and down and then in a circular movement using very light pressure. Your partner is guaranteed to find this particularly sensual.

Gently squeezing between the thumb and forefingers, work your way up on the outer part of the ears and then down inside the ears two or three times.

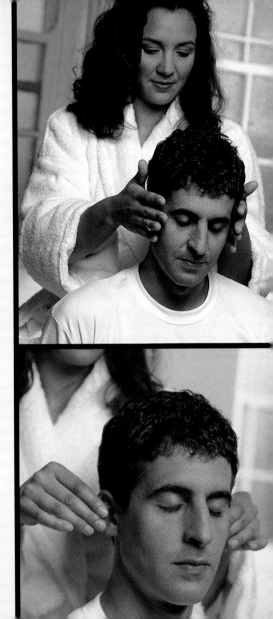

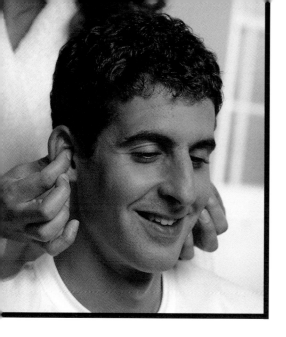

Twiddle the ears using your thumb and forefingers, covering the same area as above. Do this two or three times.

Pull the ears gently up and down.

Flick the ears.

By now your partner's ears will be red hot! He or she will feel tingly all over the ears and the face as the energy rushes down their whole body.

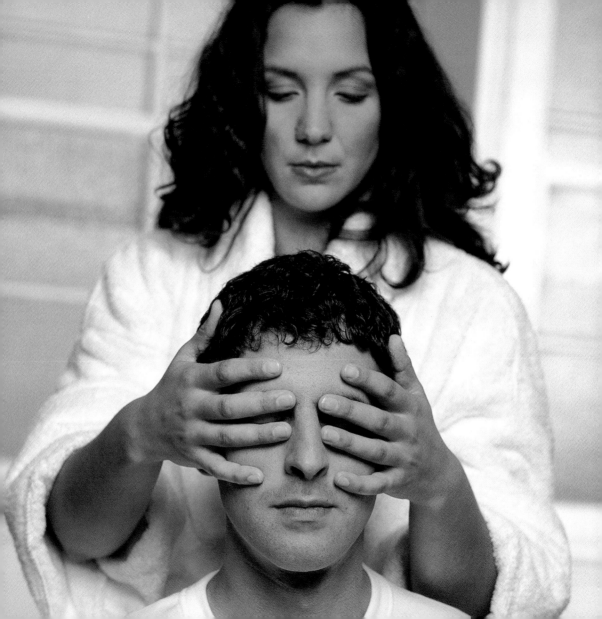

Gentle face massage

First stroke lightly up and down, and then side to side on either side of the face, using the entire surface of your hands. With the palm against the face, move slowly down from the forehead to the chin. You can repeat this movement as many times as you like.

Next, place your hands on your partner's cheeks. With your fingers facing the centre of your partner's face, hold the position for about ten seconds. Breathe calmly and deeply. Repeat the same, placing your hands on your partner's forehead. Repeat the same again, this time placing your hands on the top of your partner's head.

This massage is wonderful for leaving a tense and tired face looking beautifully relaxed and tranquil.

When you are ready to end the massage, lay your hands lightly on your partner's head in the same way as you did when you began.

Self Massage

You don't need anyone with you to experience the benefits of Indian head massage: you yourself have the power in your own fingertips to melt away pain and relieve stress. Get into the habit of giving yourself a massage at least once a week. You will find that it keeps stress at bay and replenishes vitality, leaving you refreshed and renewed, re-energized, calm and focused, easing your aching muscles and helping you to have a restful night's sleep. These simple techniques will help you to help yourself wherever and whenever you choose.

You can carry out self massage anywhere, but it is best to try and find somewhere quiet where you can be alone and concentrate on the healing power of your fingers. Make sure that the room you choose is warm and, if possible, shut the door to make sure you won't be disturbed. Wear something loose and comfortable that allows you to move your arms about freely.

I prefer to use oil with self massage, but it can still be an effective destressor without it.

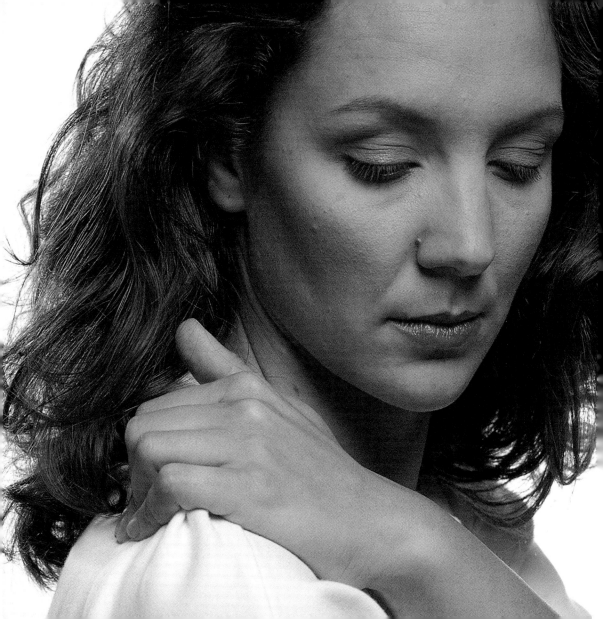

Preparing yourself

Sit with both feet on the ground, shoulders back, eyes closed, hands in your lap. Concentrate on your breathing. Try breathing deeply in and out through your nose and repeat this three times. Feel your ribcage expand as you breath in and imagine your everyday worries are being expelled with each breath out.

Keeping your eyes closed, try and visualize yourself in a warm, sunny garden. Imagine the warmth of the sun melting away the stiffness in your muscles. Then concentrate on each body part in turn. Feel your arms and hands: can you feel any pain? Imagine the pain is seeping out of your muscles and your arms are feeling heavy and warm. Next, concentrate on your shoulders: imagine the pain disappearing, leaving your shoulders smooth and flexible. Now concentrate on your head: look up and down and side to side, imagine that the stiffness is draining away, leaving the muscles warm and relaxed. Visualize your face muscles becoming soft and smooth. Try and smile and hold the smile for a few seconds. Repeat the whole sequence.

Feel that your whole body is warm and the day's tension is melting away. Concentrate again on your breathing. When you are ready, open your eyes. Stretch your arms out to the sides and then take them above your head. Stretch your body up. Now you are ready to begin.

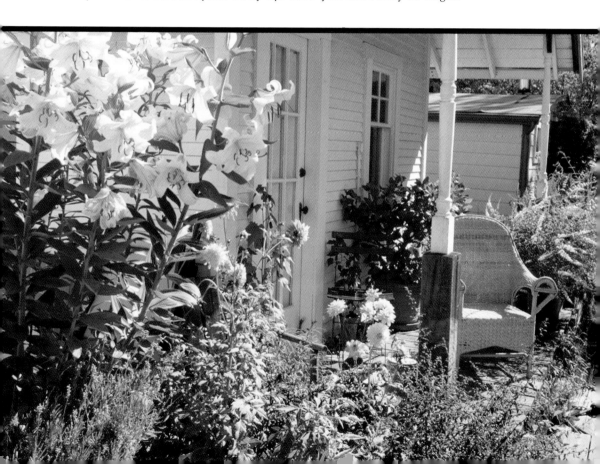

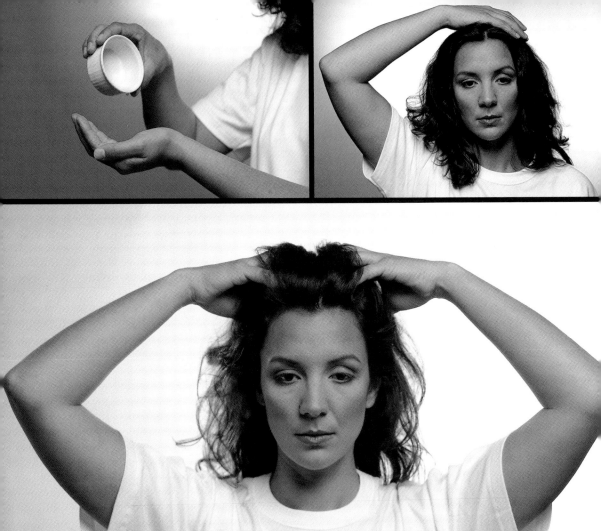

Your step-by-step guide

Pour some oil into your hand and apply it to the top of the head (on the crown). Pour some more oil into your hand and rub it between both palms.

Massage the oil into your head, starting from the sides and working towards the top. Next, work your way towards the front and back of the head, thus covering your entire head. This will distribute the oil evenly.

Now gently massage the whole of the area with your thumbs and fingers, releasing any tension by friction and rubbing.

Grasp fistfuls of hair at the roots and tug from side to side, keeping your knuckles very close to the scalp.

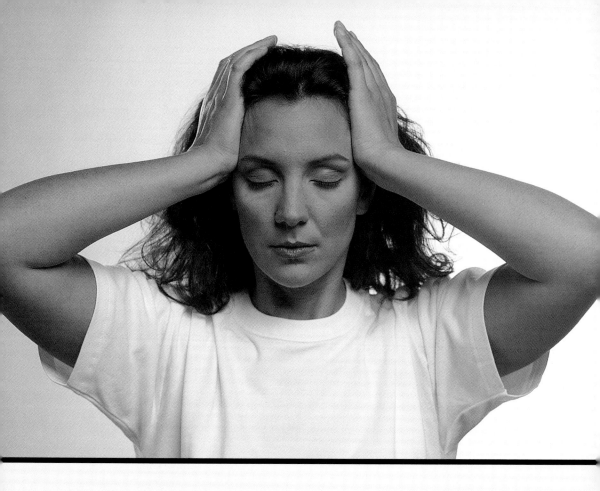

Squeeze at the temples with the heels of the hands and make slow, wide, circular movements.

Look down slightly and massage the back of the neck by squeezing and rolling the muscles. Start at the top of the neck and work your way down, first with one hand and then with the other. Repeat this a few times.

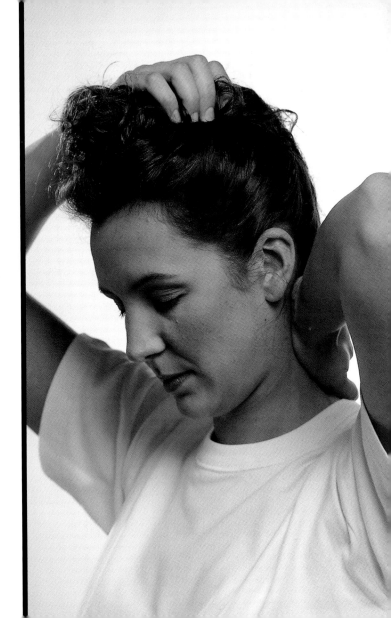

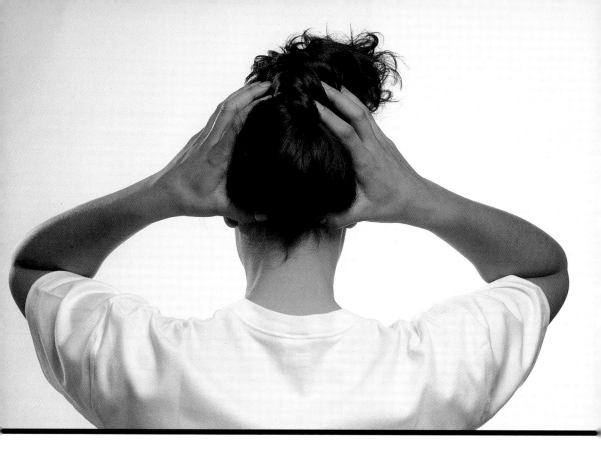

Place the thumb of your left hand under the left occipital area (base of the head) and the thumb of your right hand under the right occipital area, and relax the tight muscles by using friction or a rubbing movement.

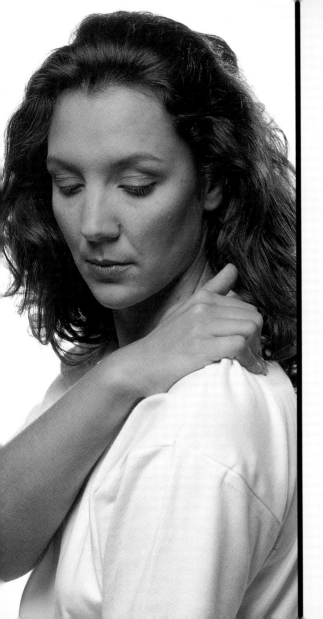

Place your right hand on your left shoulder near your neck. Using medium pressure, gently squeeze the shoulder muscle that starts at the base of your neck. Work your way outwards along your shoulder to your arm and then down as far as your elbow. When you reach your elbow, go back to the base of your neck and do this twice more. Concentrate on squeezing the muscle tissue. This squeezing technique will improve blood circulation and help to release and disperse toxins from tight muscles (you can help the removal of toxins from your body by drinking plenty of water).

Now, place the flattened palm of your right hand beside the base of your neck on the left-hand side. Rub along the top of your left shoulder and continue down your left arm where you squeezed the muscles before. When you reach your elbow, go back to the base of the neck and repeat the action twice. Change arms and work the other side. This rubbing technique will also help to release and disperse toxins from tight muscles and improve blood circulation.

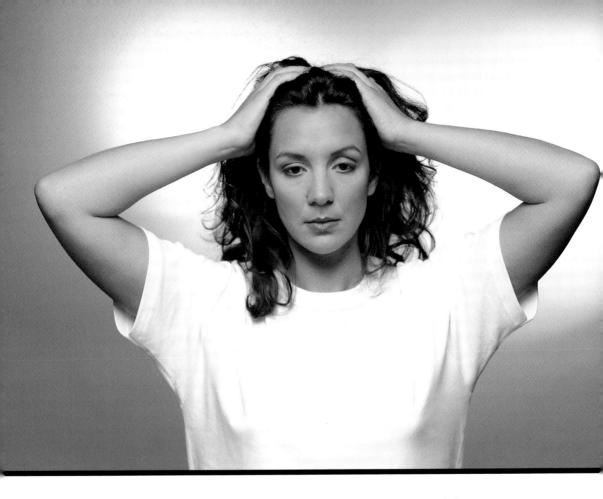

Finally, rub lightly with your hands all over the head. Extend this movement to cover your face.

If possible, always allow a few minutes after a self massage session to relax your body and mind or to carry out a few gentle stretching exercises.

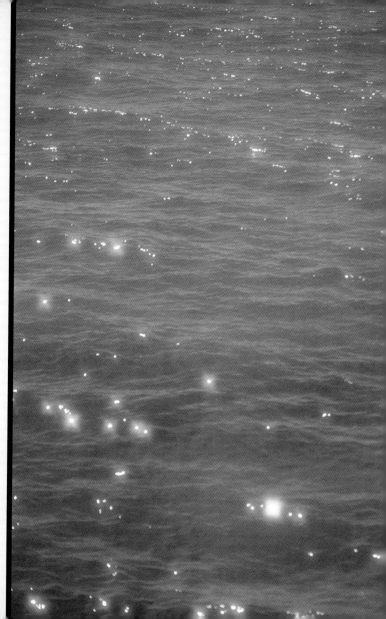

Using Oils

The incorporation of oils into Indian head massage can be very beneficial, particularly for the hair. Oil applied to the head is absorbed into the roots of the hair, strengthening it and removing dryness, which is responsible for brittle hair and some scalp disorders. Oil can soften the skin of the scalp, promote hair growth, slow down hair loss and create vibrant, shiny hair.

Choosing an oil

As the oils are partially absorbed through the pores of the skin, the best ones to use are pure organic oils.

Sesame oil

This is probably the most popular oil in India and the best general oil. It reduces swelling, relieves muscular pains and stiffness, strengthens and moisturises the skin, and is believed to keep the hair in healthy condition. It is traditionally used in the summer. It may irritate sensitive skin: if this happens, use olive oil instead.

Mustard oil

This pungent oil is one of the most popular in Northern India. It gives a warming sensation, and is effective in increasing body heat and relieving pains, swelling and stiff muscles. It helps to cleanse the blood by opening the pores and it has a general strengthening and moisturizing effect. As this oil creates a sensation of heat, it is particularly recommended for use during the winter.

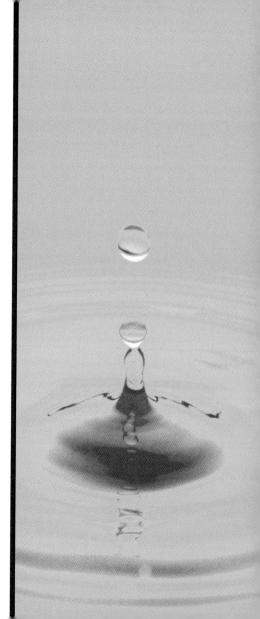

Olive oil

This is freely available in the West. It can be used on the body to relieve muscular stiffness and pain, increase body heat and reduce swelling. This is a good oil to use in the summer, and is a suitable alternative to sesame oil.

Almond oil

This is a popular massage oil in the West and is good for warming the body, reducing any pain or stiffness, and to promote healthy hair.

Coconut oil

This oil may be a little difficult to find in the West, but it is well worth the effort as it has a beautiful aroma and is a pleasure to work with. Traditionally used in the spring, coconut oil is a light oil that can help to moisturize the skin, encourage healthy hair growth, and balance the body in the process. As coconut oil is solid at room temperature, liquify it by standing it in warm water for a few minutes before use.

Applying oils

The oil should be warm – stand the bottle in a bowl of warm water for a few minutes first. If you are going to use essential oils with your massage then think ahead and have the oils ready-mixed with the top of the bottle unscrewed so that you don't break the rhythm during the course of the massage to grapple with a bottle stopper.

Both you and the person receiving the massage should choose clothes that won't be ruined if the oil gets on to them. Have a towel to hand in case of any spills.

To apply the oil, pour a few drops on to your palm and gently rub it on the top of the other person's head. Take some more oil on to your palm and then rub it between both hands and apply it to the other person's head and hair, working up towards the crown. Make sure the oil is evenly spread over the head.

Essential oils

The popularity of aromatherapy with its use of essential oils may have enjoyed a recent boom, but the properties of these oils have been appreciated for centuries. The combination of head massage and the sensual, relaxing aroma of these fragrant oils will transport the person being massaged into the realm of bliss.

For a sensual massage with your partner, choose from sandalwood, patchouli, musk, rose, jasmine, clary sage or ylang ylang. Combine two of these, or add a spicy, stimulating oil such as cardamom, ginger, cinnamon or coriander.

Essential oils are extremely concentrated and should never be used direct on the skin. Always blend them with a base oil, which could be almond, sunflower or sesame oil. Simply add a few drops of the essential oil to the base oil in a bottle and shake. Store the blended oils in pretty, dark glass bottles to enhance their look and preserve their properties.

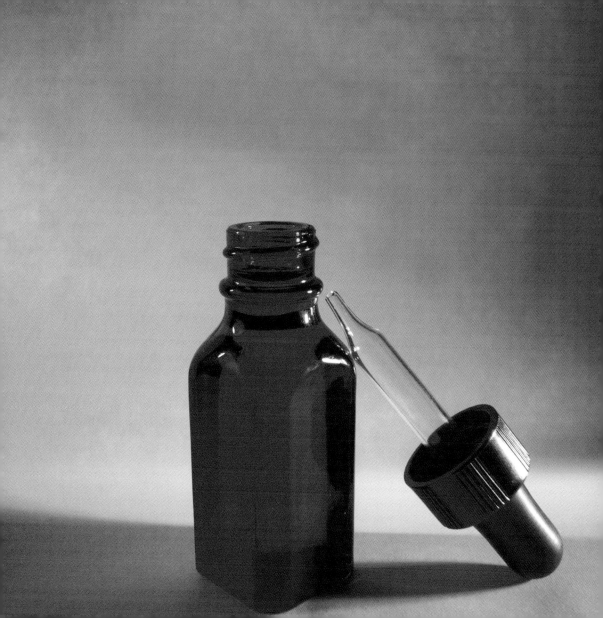

Oils for the hair

Indian women often use oil to keep their hair lustrous and strong. Regular head massage using the oil of your choice (such as olive, almond, coconut or sesame oil) is an effective way of keeping your hair in tip top condition. Essential oils can be added to these base oils to treat specific hair conditions.

Essential oils for specific hair conditions

For greasy hair	clary sage, chamomile, lemongrass
For dry/damaged hair	ylang ylang, sandalwood, rosewood
For normal hair	geranium, lavender, rosemary
For light hair	lavender, lemon
For dark hair	sandalwood, patchouli, ylang ylang
As a rinse/tonic	rosemary, petitgrain, ylang ylang
For growth	juniper, rosemary
For an itchy scalp	cedarwood, tea tree
For dandruff	patchouli, tea tree

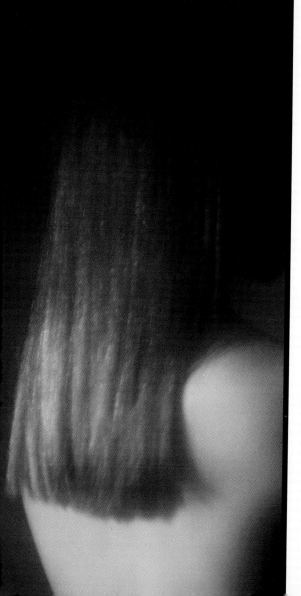

Dry or chemically treated hair

This treatment makes your hair very oily but it does have a wonderful effect. Pour 25ml olive oil, 10ml jojoba oil and 10ml wheatgerm oil into a clean bottle. Add 3ml of an essential oil blend consisting of 8 drops geranium, 12 drops lavender and 6 drops patchouli. Shake well. Apply 5–15ml of the blend to damp, but not dripping, wet hair. Rub in and leave for 20 minutes before washing your hair (you will find it easier to remove the oil if you rub a little shampoo into your hair and scalp before you wet it). Repeat twice a week for 4–6 weeks.

Dandruff

For dandruff, pour 100ml jojoba or apricot oil (or a mixture of the two) into a bottle and add the following essential oils: 20 drops orange, 17 drops cedarwood, 17 drops patchouli and 10 drops tea tree. Shake well. Massage the blend into the scalp and through the hair, taking care to keep it off the face as the mix is quite strong. Cover your hair with a towel and relax for a few hours. Shampoo and dry as normal.

Repeat twice a week if your dandruff is severe. Omit the tea tree oil and use once a week for mild dandruff.

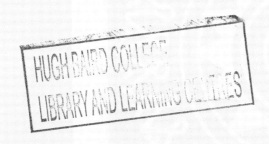